CUMULATIVE RECORD BOOK FOR GENERAL NURSING AND MIDWIFERY COURSE

CUMULATIVE RECORD BOOK FOR GENERAL NURSING AND MIDWIFERY COURSE

SECOND EDITION

R Sreevani PhD (Psychiatric Nursing)
Professor and Head
Department of Nursing
Dharwad Institute of Mental Health and Neurosciences (DIMHANS)
Dharwad, Karnataka, India

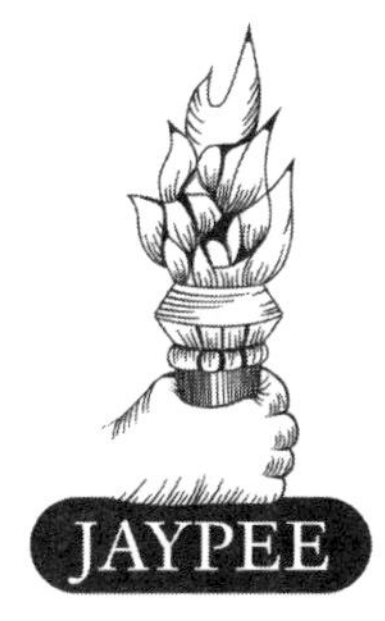

JAYPEE BROTHERS MEDICAL PUBLISHERS
The Health Sciences Publisher
New Delhi | London

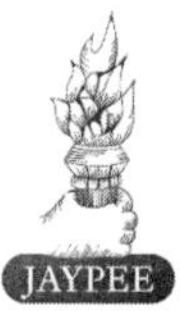

Jaypee Brothers Medical Publishers (P) Ltd

Headquarters
EMCA House, 23/23-B
Ansari Road, Daryaganj
New Delhi 110 002, India
Landline: +91-11-23272143, +91-11-23272703
+91-11-23282021, +91-11-23245672
e-mail: jaypee@jaypeebrothers.com

Corporate Office
4838/24, Ansari Road, Daryaganj
New Delhi 110 002, India
Phone: +91-11-43574357
Fax: +91-11-43574314
e-mail: jaypee@jaypeebrothers.com

Overseas Office
JP Medical Ltd.
83, Victoria Street, London
SW1H 0HW (UK)
Phone: +44-20 3170 8910
e-mail: info@jpmedpub.com

EU GPSR Authorised Representative
Logos Europe, 9 rue Nicolas Poussin
17000, La Rochelle, France
Phone: +33 (0) 6 67 93 73 78
e-mail: contact@logoseurope.eu

Website: www.jaypeebrothers.com
Website: www.jaypeedigital.com

Inquiries for bulk sales may be solicited at: jaypee@jaypeebrothers.com

Cumulative Record Book for General Nursing and Midwifery Course

First Edition: 2016

Second Edition: 2022

Reprint 2024, 2025, **2026**

ISBN 978-93-5465-157-1

Printed at: Sterling Graphics Pvt. Ltd. India

Florence Nightingale

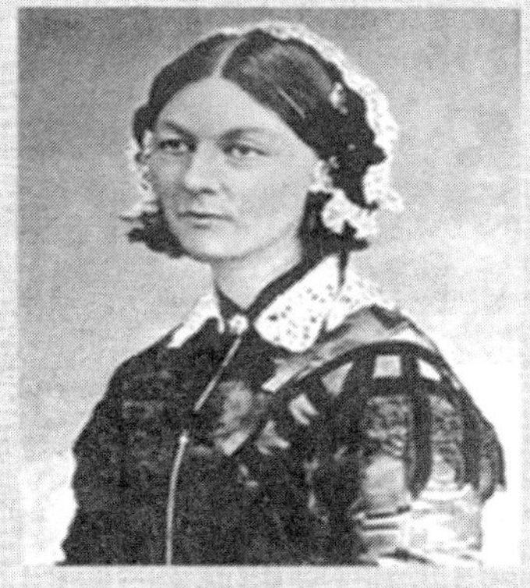

Florence Nightingale

Born: May 12, 1820 **Died:** August 13, 1910

History: Nightingale served as a nurse during the Crimean War, tending to wounded soldiers. She was called **"The Lady with the Lamp"** because of her habit of making rounds at night.

Florence Nightingale - "Founder of Modern Nursing"

She laid the foundation of professional nursing with the establishment of her nursing school at St Thomas' Hospital in London. It was the first secular nursing school in the world and is now part of King's College London. The Nightingale Pledge, taken by new nurses, was named in Florence Nightingale's honor.

Nurses Day is celebrated around the world on Florence Nightingale's birthday.

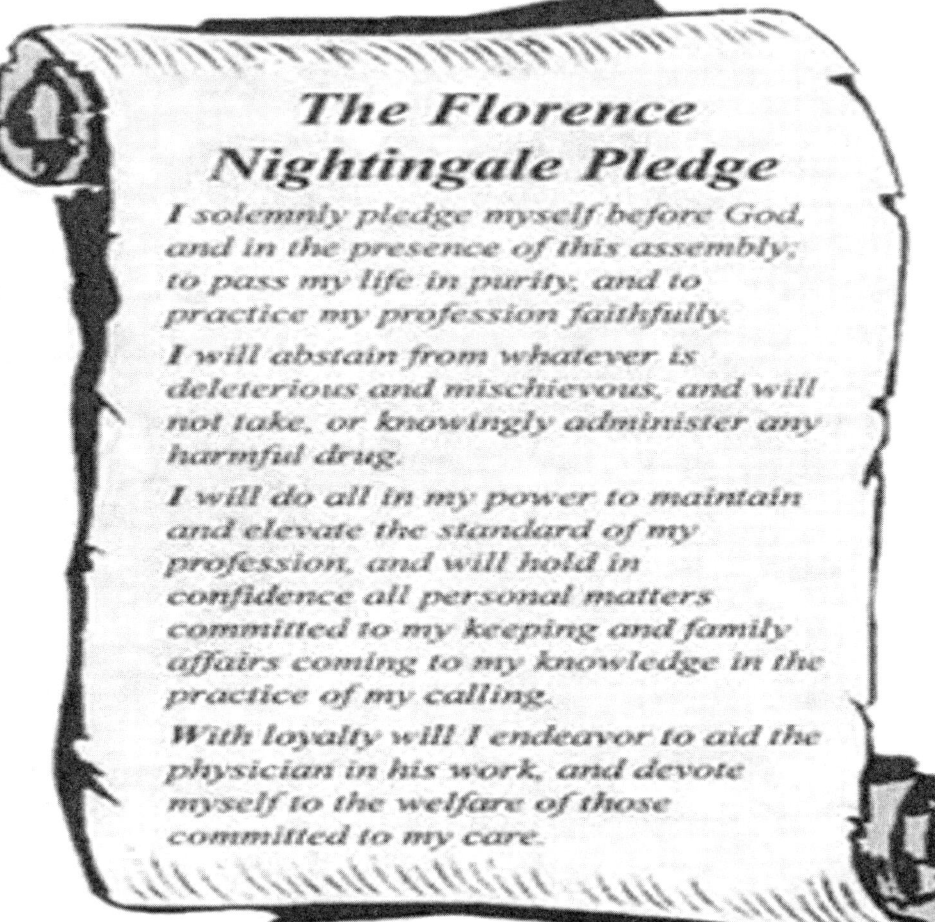

Guidelines for the use of Cumulative Record

Nursing is a combination of art and science. Each nurse practices this combination of art and science by utilizing her experience, knowledge and resources to promote the health and wellbeing of patients. It is also true that nurses are lifelong learners striving to affect positive outcomes for people and communities by providing care based on scientific principles. They are keenly aware of the uniqueness of individuals, families and communities and the need to individualize their assessment and plan of care. To meet this end, the nurse should have a thorough knowledge of all the nursing procedures. These procedures are to be learned in an organized and repetitive fashion.

The purpose of maintaining a cumulative record is to ensure that the student nurse has performed the procedures to the satisfaction of the nursing tutor/clinical instructor/ward-in-charge.

This cumulative record book presents a list of nursing procedures both year wise and subject wise for General nursing and Midwifery students. It is written methodically as per the revised Indian Nursing Council (INC) syllabus 2015. It will aid the students in getting beforehand information of the procedures they will be required to perform. It is a written document for the student as well as the teacher.

The cumulative record book has been organized as under:

- Guidelines for clinical evaluation
- Year wise list of assignments to be completed (including care plan and case presentations)
- List of procedures to be performed by the nursing student with columns for marking date of demonstration and return demonstration
- Year wise examination result sheet for noting attendance percentage, internal and board examination marks

The student should be given an opportunity to practice in the clinical area as early as possible following the laboratory demonstration. Once the student acquires adequate skills in performing the procedure the respective date may be marked by the tutor.

After completion the record book is scrutinized by subject teachers, class coordinator and the principal. The student is then certified as eligible for taking up the final examination. During the state board examination, the examiners shall check for completion of performance of all procedures. Signatures of the internal and external examiners are to be obtained in respective places.

TABLE OF CONTENTS

STUDENT PROFILE

PHOTOGRAPH

Name of the Institution : ____________________

Address of the Institution : ____________________

____

Name of the student : ____________________

(in block letters)

Reg. No. : ____________________

Date of birth : ____________________

Age in years : ____________________

Father's name : ____________________

Residential address : ____

____

Date of joining the course : ____________________

Date of completing the course : ____________________

Identification marks : 1. ____________________

2. ____________________

Signature of the student

Date:

Signature of the principal

Date:

GENERAL NURSING AND MIDWIFERY COURSE

Duration: 3 years

GUIDELINES FOR CLINICAL/FIELD WORK EVALUATION

1. There shall be 50% internal assessment for all the practical examinations.
2. A regular and periodic assessment for each subject and clinical/field experience is to be carried out.
3. For the purpose of internal assessment a subject wise written test shall be conducted every month.
4. The student shall be required to maintain a:
   - Practical record book
   - Report of observation visits
   - Daily diary for assessment
5. Marks shall be allotted for each of the following:
   - Case study
   - Case presentation
   - Nursing care plan
   - Maintenance of record books (Procedure Book and Midwifery Record book)
   - Daily diary
6. Area wise clinical assessment is to be carried out (minimum two assessments are required in each clinical area).
7. A candidate must secure at least 50% marks in each of the theory and practical internal assessments.
8. If a candidate fails in either theory or practical paper he/she will have to re-appear for both the papers (theory and practical).

FIRST YEAR

DETAILS OF COURSE INSTRUCTION (THEORY AND PRACTICAL)

Sl. No.	*Subjects*	*Hours prescribed by INC*	*Completed hours*	*Name of the teacher*	*Teacher signature*
		THEORY			
1.	Biosciences • Anatomy and physiology • Microbiology	**120** 90 30			
2.	Behavioral sciences • Psychology • Sociology	**60** 40 20			
3.	Nursing foundation • Fundamentals of nursing • First aid	**210** 190 20			
4.	Community health nursing • Community health nursing – 1 • Environmental hygiene • Health education and communication skills • Nutrition	**180** 80 30 40 30			
5.	English	30			
6.	Computer education	15			
7.	Co-curricular activities	10			
	Total Hours (Weeks)	**625 (16)**			
		PRACTICAL			
1.	Nursing foundation	200 laboratory + 680 clinicals (22 weeks)			
	a. Name of the hospital				
	Names of the wards • • • •				
2.	Community health nursing	320 (8 weeks)			
	a. Name of the community area				
	b. Names of the PHC/CHC				
3.	Computer education	15			
	Total Hours (Weeks)	**1215 (30)**			

LIST OF FIRST YEAR ASSIGNMENTS

a. Nursing care plan: 4 in medical/surgical wards
b. Daily diary: 1 each in urban and rural community field
c. Health talk: 1 each in urban and rural community field
d. Family study: 1 each in urban and rural community field
e. Health assessment of an individual in the family: 1 each in urban and rural community field
f. Community profile: 1 each in urban and rural community field

NURSING FOUNDATION PRACTICAL

Placement: I Year—Practical Hours (880 hours): 200 Laboratory hours + 680 Clinical hours

Procedure	*Date of demonstration*	*Teacher signature*	*Date of return demonstration*	*Supervisor signature*
1. **Hospital admission**				
1.1. Preparation of unit for new patient				
1.2. Preparation of admission bed				
1.3. Admission procedure for new patient				
1.4. Admission procedure for transfer in patient				
1.5. Record of admission procedure				
2. **Discharge/transfer out**				
2.1. Discharge counseling				
2.2. Discharge procedure for planned discharge				
2.3. Discharge procedure for leaving against medical advice (LAMA)				
2.4. Discharge procedure for referrals and transfers				
2.5. Discharge procedure for transfer in patient				
2.6. Record of discharge procedure				
2.7. Disinfection of unit and equipment after discharge/ transfer				
3. **Nursing assessment and interventions for patients**				
3.1. History taking				
3.2. Nursing diagnosis				
3.3. Listing nursing problems				
3.4. Prioritization of problems				
3.5. Goals and expected outcomes				
3.6. Nursing interventions				
3.7. Evaluation				
3.8. Writing nursing care plan				
3.9. Providing care as per the plan				
4. **Communication**				
4.1. Use of verbal and non-verbal communication techniques				
5. **Prepare a plan for patient teaching session**				
5.1. Develop plan for patient teaching				
5.2. Provide health talk				
6. **Write patient report**				
6.1. Change of shift reports				
6.2. Transfer reports				
6.3. Incident reports				
6.4. Oral report presentation				
6.5. Daily care planning/time planning				
7. **Vital signs**				
7.1. Temperature ◆ Oral ◆ Auxillary ◆ Rectum				

Procedure	Date of demonstration	Teacher signature	Date of return demonstration	Supervisor signature
7.2. Pulse				
7.3. Respiration				
7.4. Blood pressure				
7.5. Temperature, pulse, respiration (TPR) recording				
8. **Health assessment**				
8.1. History taking				
8.2. Perform physical examination ◆ Inspection ◆ Palpation ◆ Percussion ◆ Auscultation ◆ Olfaction				
8.3. Identification of system wise deviations				
8.4. Pain assessment				
9. **Preparation of patient's unit**				
9.1. Open bed				
9.2. Closed bed				
9.3. Occupied bed				
9.4. Operation bed				
9.5. Cardiac bed				
9.6. Fracture bed				
9.7. Burn bed				
9.8. Divided and Fowler's bed				
9.9. Amputation bed				
9.10. Digitally operated beds				
10. **Provision for comfort devices**				
10.1. Mattress (air, water)				
10.2. Extra pillows				
10.3. Back rest				
10.4. Cardiac table				
10.5. Bed cradle				
10.6. Air cushion				
10.7. Foot rest				
10.8. Cotton rings, hand rolls, pads				
10.9. Hot water bottles				
10.10. Trochanter rolls				
10.11. Sand bags				
11. **Hygienic care**				
11.1. Oral hygiene for unconscious patient				
11.2. Assisting for oral hygiene				
11.3. Bed bath				
11.4. Assisted bath/bathroom bath				
11.5. Back care				
11.6. Care of pressure points				
11.7. Hair combing				
11.8. Hair wash				

Procedure	Date of demonstration	Teacher signature	Date of return demonstration	Supervisor signature
11.9. Pediculosis treatment				
11.10. Care of nails—hand and feet				
12. Feeding				
12.1. Oral feeding				
12.2. Naso/orogastric feeding				
12.3. Gastrostomy feeding				
12.4. Parenteral feeding				
12.5. Nasogastric tube insertion				
12.6. Nasogastric tube suction				
12.7. Nasogastric tube irrigation				
13. Urinary elimination				
13.1. Provide urinal/bed pan				
13.2. Condom drainage				
13.3. Perineal care				
13.4. Catheterization				
13.5. Care of urinary drainage				
13.6. Bladder irrigation				
14. Bowel elimination				
14.1. Insertion of flatus tube				
14.2. Cleansing enema				
14.3. Insertion of suppository				
14.4. Assist for medicated packs into rectum				
14.5. Bowel wash				
15. Body alignment and mobility				
15.1. Range of motion exercises • Active exercises • Passive exercises				
15.2. Deep breathing and coughing exercises				
15.3. Supine position				
15.4. Dorsal recumbent position				
15.5. Lateral/side lying position				
15.6. Prone position				
15.7. Fowler's/semi Fowler's position				
15.8. C-position				
15.9. Sims position				
15.10. Lithotomy position				
15.11. Trendelenburg position				
15.12. Assisting the patient in changing position				
15.13. Assisting the patient for sitting position				
15.14. Assisting the patient in transferring from bed to wheel chair				
15.15. Assisting the patient in transferring from bed to stretcher				
15.16. Assisting the patient in walking				
15.17. Helping the patient with the crutches				
15.18. Helping the patient with the walker				

Procedure	Date of demonstration	Teacher signature	Date of return demonstration	Supervisor signature
15.19. Application of restraints				
15.20. Care of patient with restraints				
16. Oxygen administration				
16.1. Preparation for oxygen administration				
16.2. Oxygen administration ◆ Mask ◆ Prongs ◆ Tent ◆ Catheters				
16.3. Care of oxygen cylinder				
17. Suctioning				
17.1. Arranging suction equipment				
17.2. Oropharyngeal				
17.3. Nasopharyngeal				
18. Chest physiotherapy and postural drainage				
18.1. Care of chest drainage				
18.2. Chest physiotherapy ◆ Postural drainage ◆ Chest percussion ◆ Vibration				
19. Cardiopulmonary resuscitation (CPR)—Basic life support				
19.1. Cardiopulmonary resuscitation				
20. Intravenous therapy				
20.1. Observation of IV therapy				
20.2. Observation of blood and blood component transfusion				
20.3. Maintenance of intake and output chart				
21. Collection of specimens for investigation				
21.1. Urine ◆ Routine ◆ Culture ◆ 24 hours				
21.2. Sputum				
21.3. Feces				
21.4. Vomitus				
21.5. Blood				
21.6. Vaginal discharge				
21.7. Peripheral smear				
21.8. Throat swab				
22. Perform laboratory test				
22.1. Urine for sugar				
22.2. Urine for albumin				
22.3. Urine for acetone				
22.4. Urine for specific gravity				
22.5. Urine for bile pigments and salts				
22.6. Blood for sugar (with strip/glucometer)				
23. Application of hot and cold therapies				
23.1. Hot water bag				
23.2. Hot fomentation				

Procedure	Date of demonstration	Teacher signature	Date of return demonstration	Supervisor signature
23.3. Infrared/ultra violet lamp				
23.4. Steam inhalation				
23.5. Dry cold application/ice cap				
23.6. Moist cold application/cold sponging/tepid sponging				
23.7. Sitz bath				
24. **Communication and assisting with special population**				
24.1. Assisting with self-care of visually impaired patient				
24.2. Assisting with self-care of hearing impaired patient				
24.3. Communicating with visually impaired patient				
24.4. Communicating with hearing impaired patient				
24.5. Communicating with mentally disturbed patient				
24.6. Assisting with self-care of mentally disturbed patient				
24.7. Assisting with self-care of mentally challenged individual				
25. **Recreational and diversional therapies**				
25.1. Providing recreational and diversional therapies to patients				
26. **Care of patient with alteration in sensorium**				
26.1. Assessment of patient with alteration in sensorium				
26.2. Care of patient with alteration in sensorium				
27. **Infection control**				
27.1. Medical hand washing				
27.2. Surgical hand washing (scrub)				
27.3. Preparing isolation unit				
27.4. Wearing and removal of mask				
27.5. Wearing and removal of gloves				
27.6. Wearing and removal of gown				
27.7. Practice technique of wearing and removing of personal protective equipment (donning and doffing of PPE)				
27.8. Practice standard of safety precautions				
28. **Disinfection of equipment and unit—sterilization**				
28.1. Boiling method				
28.2. Autoclaving				
28.3. Hot air oven				
28.4. Chemical method				
28.5. Mechanical method				
28.6. Handling sterilized equipment				
28.7. Calculation of strength of lotions				
28.8. Preparation of lotions				
28.9. Care of rubber goods				
28.10. Care of soiled linen				
28.11. Care of mattress and pillows				
28.12. Care of enamel goods				
28.13. Care of needles				
28.14. Care of sharp instruments				

Procedure	Date of demonstration	Teacher signature	Date of return demonstration	Supervisor signature
29. **Biomedical waste management**				
29.1. Decontamination of hospital waste				
29.2. Segregation and transportation of waste				
30. **Care of wound**				
30.1. Skin preparation for surgery (local)				
30.2. Preparation of postoperative unit				
30.3. Preoperative teaching and counseling				
30.4. Postoperative teaching and counseling				
30.5. Pre and postoperative monitoring of patient				
30.6. Wound dressing				
30.7. Care of wound drainage				
30.8. Application of abdominal binders				
30.9. Application of breast binders				
30.10. Application of T-binders				
31. **Bandages for various body parts**				
31.1. Application of splints				
31.2. Application of slings				
31.3. Application of circular bandage				
31.4. Application of spiral bandage				
31.5. Application of spiral reverse bandage				
31.6. Application of figure-of-eight bandage				
31.7. Application of capeline bandage				
31.8. Application of eye bandage				
31.9. Application of jaw bandage				
31.10. Application of ear bandage				
31.11. Application of shoulder spica bandage				
31.12. Application of triangular bandage				
31.13. Preparation of first-aid kit				
32. **Administration of medications in different forms and routes**				
32.1. Oral				
32.2. Sublingual				
32.3. Intradermal				
32.4. Subcutaneous				
32.5. Intramuscular				
32.6. Intravenous				
32.7. Drug measurement and dose calculation				
32.8. Preparation of lotions and solutions				
33. **Administration of topical applications, insertion of drug into body cavity**				
33.1. Insertion of suppository and medicated packs				
33.2. Instillation of ear drops				
33.3. Instillation of eye drops				
33.4. Instillation of nose drops				
33.5. Instillation of throat drops				
33.6. Irrigation of eye				
33.7. Irrigation of ear				

Procedure	*Date of demonstration*	*Teacher signature*	*Date of return demonstration*	*Supervisor signature*
33.8. Irrigation of bladder				
33.9. Irrigation of vagina				
33.10. Irrigation of rectum				
34. **Inhalations**				
34.1. Dry inhalations				
34.2. Moist inhalations				
34.3. Plain nebulization				
34.4. Medicated nebulization				
34.5. Identification of spurious drugs				
34.6. Recording of medicine administration (date, time, medication, dose, route and signature)				
35. **Care of dying patient**				
35.1. Care for terminally ill patient				
35.2. Care of dead body				
35.3. Packing of dead body				
35.4. Counseling of grieving relatives				
35.5. Handing over the body to relatives				
35.6. Handing over the patient's valuables to relatives				
35.7. Transferring the dead body to mortuary				
35.8. Terminal care of the unit				

Nursing Care Plan Performed in the Hospital

Sl. No.	Date	Details of care plan	Ward	Teacher signature
1.				
2.				
3.				
4.				

Health Talks/Health Education Given in the Hospital

Sl. No.	Date	Place	Topic	Group/individual	AV aids used	Supervisor signature
1.						
2.						

Attendance in percentage (%):
Theory:
Practical:

Subject teachers **Class coordinator** **Principal**

1.
2.
3.
4.

NURSING FOUNDATION PRACTICAL EXAMINATION

Signature of internal examiner **Signature of external examiner**

Date: **Date:**

Signature of internal examiner **Signature of external examiner**

Date: **Date:**

Signature of internal examiner **Signature of external examiner**

Date: **Date:**

COMMUNITY HEALTH NURSING – I

Placement: I Year—Practical Hours: 336 (8 Weeks)

Procedure	*Date of demonstration*	*Teacher signature*	*Date of return demonstration*	*Supervisor signature*
1. Mapping of the field area ➢ Rural ➢ Urban				
2. Community health survey in rural area				
3. Community health survey in urban area				
4. Identification of community needs				
5. Organization and conduct of home visits				
6. Build up and maintain rapport with family				
7. Demonstrate bag technique				
8. Assessment of family environment ➢ Housing/sanitary condition				
9. Health assessment of family				
10. Nutritional assessment of individuals				
11. Identification of health needs ➢ Infant ➢ Toddler ➢ Pre-schooler ➢ School age child ➢ Adolescent ➢ Adult ➢ Old age person				
12. Listing the health needs of the family				
13. Providing care at home as per standing orders				
14. Demonstrating different methods of preparing food according to the nutritionals needs of the family				
15. Making referrals				
16. Planning and conducting individual health education on identified needs				
17. Planning and conducting group health education				
18. Maintaining family folders				
19. Assisting for set-up of clinics in the community				
20. Collection and recording of vital health statistics				
21. Administration of medications in: ➢ Subcenter ➢ Primary Health center ➢ Community Health center				
22. Assisting for immunization activities				
23. Maintenance of records and reports				
23.1. Birth and death registers				
23.2. Immunization registers				
23.3. Antenatal and postnatal registers				
23.4. Family planning register				
23.5. Stock register				
24. Treatment for minor ailments				

Assignments Performed in the Community

Sl. No.	Name of the assignment	Date	Area/house address	Supervisor signature
1.	Health talk (topic name) 1. 2.			
2.	Family care plan (name of the family) 1. 2.			
3.	Health assessment of individual (name of the individual) 1. 2.			
4.	Community profile (name of the community) 1. 2.			
5.	Daily diary	Submission date:		

Observational Report of Field Visits

Sl. No.	Date	Visit	institution address	Supervisor signature
1.		Water purification plant		
2.		Sewage treatment plant		
3.		Milk dairy		
4.		Food processing unit		
5.		Gram panchayat		
6.		Primary health center		
7.		Central sterile services department (CSSD)		

Attendance in percentage (%):
Theory:
Practical:

Subject teachers **Class coordinator** **Principal**

1.
2.
3.

NUTRITION PRACTICAL

Placement: I Year—Practical Hours: 8

Procedure	*Date of demonstration*	*Teacher signature*	*Date of return demonstration*	*Supervisor signature*
1. Preparation of diet—beverages				
1.1. Hot and cold				
1.2. Juice				
1.3. Shakes				
1.4. Soups				
1.5. Lassi				
1.6. Barley water				
2. Egg preparation				
2.1. Egg flip				
2.2. Scramble				
2.3. Omlet				
2.4. Poached egg				
3. Light diet				
3.1. Porridges				
3.2. Gruel				
3.3. Khichdi				
3.4. Kanji				
3.5. Boiled vegetables				
3.6. Salads				
3.7. Custard				
4. Low cost high nutrition diets				
4.1. Chikki				
4.2. Multigrain roti				

Observational Visits

Sl. No.	*Date*	*Visit*	*Institution address*	*Supervisor signature*
1.		Food processing unit		

Assignments

Sl. No.	*Assignment*	*Date*	*Supervisor signature*
1.	Preparation of charts		
2.	Conducting nutrition exhibition		

FIRST YEAR EXAMINATION RESULTS

Name of the student: Month and year of passing:

Register No.:

Hall ticket No.:

Subject	*Type of assessment*	*Max. Marks*	*Marks obtained in first attempt*	*Marks obtained in second attempt*	*Marks obtained in third attempt*
PAPER–I Anatomy, physiology and microbiology	Internal	25			
	Board/Council	75			
	Total	**100**			
PAPER–II Psychology and sociology	Internal	25			
	Board/Council	75			
	Total	**100**			
PAPER–III Fundamentals of nursing and first aid	Internal	25			
	Board/Council	75			
	Total	**100**			
PAPER–IV Community health nursing	Internal	25			
	Board/Council	75			
	Total	**100**			
PRACTICAL–I Fundamentals of nursing	Internal	50			
	Board/Council	50			
	Total	**100**			

Note: Minimum pass percentage—50% in each subject

SECOND YEAR

DETAILS OF COURSE INSTRUCTION (THEORY AND PRACTICAL)

Sl. No.	*Subjects*	*Hours prescribed by INC*	*Completed hours*	*Name of the teacher*	*Teacher signature*
		THEORY			
1.	Medical surgical nursing – I	120			
2.	Medical surgical nursing – II	120			
3.	Mental health nursing	70			
4.	Child health nursing	70			
5.	Co-curricular activities	20			
	Total Hours (Weeks)	**400 (10)**			
		PRACTICAL			
1.	Medical surgical nursing – I	800 (20 weeks)			
2.	Medical surgical nursing – II				
3.	Mental health nursing	320 (8 weeks)			
4.	Child health nursing	320 (8 weeks)			
	Total Hours (Weeks)	**1440 (36)**			

LIST OF SECOND YEAR ASSIGNMENTS

Medical ward	*Surgical ward*	*Psychiatry ward*	*Pediatric ward*
• Nursing care plan—2 • Case study—1 • Case presentation—1 • Drug study—1	• Nursing care plan—2 • Case study—1 • Case presentation—1 • Drug study—1	• Nursing care plan—1 • Case study—1 • Case presentation—1 • Drug study—1 • Process recording—2 • History taking—4 • Mental status examination—4	• Nursing care plan—2 • Case study—1 • Case presentation—1 • Drug study—1 • Observation report (newborn)—2

MEDICAL SURGICAL NURSING - I

Placement: II Year—Clinical Hours: 800 (20 Weeks)

Procedure	*Date of demonstration*	*Teacher signature*	*Date of return demonstration*	*Supervisor signature*
Medical wards (Resp, GI, Endo, Hemato, Neuro, Renal)—3 weeks duration				
1. **Assessment of patient**				
1.1. History taking				
1.2. Physical examination—general and specific				
1.3. Identifying alterations/deviations				
2. **Practice medical-surgical asepsis**				
2.1. Medical asepsis				
2.2. Surgical asepsis				
2.3. Safety measures				
3. **Administer medications**				
3.1. Oral				
3.2. Sublingual				
3.3. Intradermal				
3.4. Subcutaneous				
3.5. Intramuscular				
3.6. Intravenous				
3.7. Total parental nutrition				
3.8. Dosage calculation				
4. **Intravenous therapy**				
4.1. Insertion of IV cannula				
4.2. Maintenance and monitoring				
5. **Oxygen therapy**				
5.1. Mask				
5.2. Nasal cannula				
5.3. Prongs and tent				
5.4. Hood				
5.5. Steam inhalation				
5.6. Nebulization				
5.7. Chest physiotherapy				
5.8. Nasogastric feeding				
6. **Assist and prepare for common diagnostic procedures**				
6.1. Electrocardiogram				
6.2. X-ray				
6.3. Scanning and ultrasound				
6.4. Echocardiogram				
6.5. Angiography				
6.6. Magnetic resonance imaging (MRI)				
6.7. Lumbar puncture				
6.8. Sternal puncture				
6.9. Renal biopsy				
6.10. Cystoscopy				
6.11. Liver biopsy				

Procedure	*Date of demonstration*	*Teacher signature*	*Date of return demonstration*	*Supervisor signature*
6.12. Laryngoscopy				
6.13. Bronchoscopy				
6.14. Barium meal				
6.15. Barium enema				
6.16. Endoscopy				
6.17. Esophagogastroduodenoscopy				
6.18. Laparoscopy				
6.19. Cholecystography				
6.20. Proctoscopy				
7. Perform/assist in therapeutic procedure				
7.1. Phlebotomy/venous puncture				
7.2. Abdominal paracentesis				
7.3. Thoracentesis				
7.4. Gastric lavage				
7.5. Intercostals tube insertion				
7.6. Water seal drainage				
7.7. Colostomy dressing				
7.8. Hemodialysis				
7.9. Peritoneal dialysis				
8. Therapeutic procedures				
8.1. Transfusion of blood and its components				
8.2. Throat suctioning				
8.3. Endotracheal tube (ET) suctioning				
8.4. Catheterization				
9. Collecting specimens for common investigations				
9.1. Urine				
9.2. Blood				
9.3. Sputum				
9.4. Feces				
9.5. Vomitus				
9.6. Vaginal discharge				
9.7. Peripheral smear				
9.8. Throat swab				
10. Maintain elimination				
10.1. Catheterization				
10.2. Condom drainage				
10.3. Care of urinary bag				
10.4. Maintain intake and output chart				
11. Education and counseling				
11.1. Educating and counseling patient regarding specific disease condition				
11.2. Educating and counseling family regarding specific disease condition				

Procedure	Date of demonstration	Teacher signature	Date of return demonstration	Supervisor signature
Surgical wards (GI and urinary)—3 weeks duration				
12. **Practice medical-surgical asepsis**				
12.1. Medical asepsis				
12.2. Surgical asepsis				
12.3. Safety measures				
13. **Preoperative care**				
13.1. Preoperative teaching				
13.2. Preoperative preparation				
14. **Postoperative care**				
14.1. Unit preparation				
14.2. Receiving the patient from OT				
14.3. Immediate assessment				
14.4. Monitoring				
14.5. Immediate postoperative care				
14.6. Care in recovery room				
14.7. Care in surgical ward				
14.8. Care of wound and dressing				
14.9. Care of drainage				
14.10. Suture removal				
14.11. Postoperative exercises				
14.12. Ambulation				
14.13. Nasogastric aspiration				
14.14. Care of chest drainage				
14.15. Ostomy care				
14.16. Gastrostomy				
14.17. Enterostomy				
14.18. Colostomy				
14.19. Transfusion of blood and its components				
Operation theater—3 weeks duration				
15. Scrubbing				
16. Gowning				
17. Gloving				
18. Identifying instruments for common operations				
19. Identifying suture material for common operations				
20. Carbolization				
21. Sterilization and fumigation				
22. Preparation and packing of instruments for surgery				
23. Setting up sterile trolley				
24. Preparing the OT table				
25. Positioning and monitoring the patient				
26. Assisting with minor surgeries 1. 2. 3. 4. 5.				

Procedure	Date of demonstration	Teacher signature	Date of return demonstration	Supervisor signature
27. Assisting with major surgeries 1. 2. 3. 4. 5.				
28. Handling specimens				
29. Segregation and disposal of biomedical waste as per guidelines				
Intensive care unit (ICU)—1 week duration				
30. Connecting and monitoring ECG				
31. Connecting and monitoring pulse oximetry				
32. Assisting in endotracheal intubation				
33. Assisting in endotracheal suctioning				
34. Care of tracheostomy patient				
35. Providing care for a patient on ventilator				
36. Handling emergency drug trolley/crash cart				
37. Assisting in insertion of central line				
38. Monitoring central venous pressure				
39. Endotracheal (ET) suctioning				
40. Oxygen administration				
Geriatric nursing—medical/surgical/special ward—1 week duration				
41. Identifying health problems among elderly				
41.1. Physiological needs				
41.2. Psychological needs				
41.3. Social needs				
41.4. Spiritual needs				
42. Implementation of care				
43. Health promotion of elderly				

MEDICAL SURGICAL NURSING - II

Placement: II Year

Procedure	*Date of demonstration*	*Teacher signature*	*Date of return demonstration*	*Supervisor signature*
Oncology ward—1 week duration				
1. **Screen for common cancers**				
1.1. Screen for tumor node metastasis				
2. **Assist and prepare for diagnostic procedures**				
2.1. Biopsies				
2.2. Pap smear				
2.3. Bone marrow				
2.4. Mammography				
3. **Assist and prepare for therapeutic procedures**				
3.1. Radiation therapy				
3.2. Chemotherapy				
4. **Observe various modalities of treatment**				
4.1. Chemotherapy				
4.2. Radiation therapy				
4.3. Pain management				
4.4. Stoma care				
4.5. Hormonal therapy				
4.6. Stem cell therapy				
4.7. Immuno therapy				
4.8. Complementary and alternative therapies				
5. Participation in palliative care				
6. Providing care for patient with cancer				
7. Teaching and counseling family members regarding disease condition				
8. Teaching and counseling patient regarding disease condition				
Dermatology and burns—1 week duration				
9. **Assessment of the burns patient**				
9.1. Assessment of percentage of burns				
9.2. Degree of burns				
10. **Fluid and electrolyte replacement therapy**				
10.1. Assess				
10.2. Calculate				
10.3. Replace				
10.4. Record				
10.5. Maintaining intake and output chart				
11. Assessment of patient with dermatological disorder				
12. Care of patient with dermatological disorder				
13. Administering topical medications				
14. Giving medicated baths				
15. Observe/assist skin grafting				
16. Performing active and passive exercises				

Procedure	*Date of demonstration*	*Teacher signature*	*Date of return demonstration*	*Supervisor signature*
17. Teaching and counseling family members regarding disease condition				
18. Teaching and counseling patient regarding disease condition				
Ophthalmology—1 week duration				
19. Perform examination of eye				
20. Assist with diagnostic procedures				
20.1. Vision test				
20.2. Tonometry				
21. Assist with therapeutic procedures				
21.1. Perform/assist with eye irrigation				
21.2. Assist for removal of foreign bodies from eye				
22. Apply eye drops/ointment				
23. Apply eye bandage				
24. Care of patient with ophthalmic problems				
24.1. Prepare the patient for ophthalmic surgeries				
24.2. Preoperative care for patients with eye surgery				
24.3. Postoperative care for patients with eye surgery				
24.4. Providing care for patients with ophthalmic problems				
25. Teach and counsel family members regarding disease condition				
26. Teach and counsel patient regarding disease condition				
Ear, nose, throat ward—1 week duration				
27. Perform examination of ear, nose, throat				
28. Assist with diagnostic procedures				
28.1. Ear function test				
28.2. Throat examination				
28.3. Collection of throat swab				
29. Assist/perform with therapeutic procedures				
29.1. Instill drops in nose				
29.2. Instill drops in ears				
29.3. Irrigation of ear				
29.4. Irrigation of nose				
29.5. Removal of foreign bodies from ear				
29.6. Removal of foreign bodies from nose				
29.7. Apply ear bandage				
29.8. Perform tracheostomy care				
30. Health education to patient and family members				
Cardiology ward/ ICCU/cardiothoracic and vascular unit—2 weeks duration				
31. Perform cardiovascular assessment				
32. Record ECG				
33. Monitor patients on cardiac monitor				
34. Monitor central venous pressure				

Procedure	*Date of demonstration*	*Teacher signature*	*Date of return demonstration*	*Supervisor signature*
35. **Prepare/assist the patient for diagnostic procedures**				
35.1. Noninvasive procedures (echo and stress test)				
35.2. Invasive procedure (angiogram)				
36. Prepare/assist the patient for therapeutic procedures				
37. Administer cardiac drugs				
38. Advanced/basic cardiac life support (ACLS/BLS)				
39. Monitor and care for patient with chest drainage				
40. Monitor patients in ICU				
41. Assist in defibrillation				
42. Maintain flow sheet				
43. Perform endotracheal suctioning				
44. Monitor and provide care for patient on ventilators				
45. Collect specimens for arterial blood gas (ABG) analysis				
46. Assist with arterial puncture				
47. Maintain central venous pressure (CVP) line				
48. Connect and monitor pulse oximetry				
49. Monitor and provide care of patient on ventilator				
50. Assist for defibrillation				
51. Assist for bag mask ventilation				
52. Maintain flowchart				
53. Prepare emergency trolley/tray/crash cart				
54. **Administer drugs**				
54.1. Infusion pump				
54.2. Epidural				
54.3. Intrathecal				
54.4. Intracardiac				
55. Assist for total parental therapy				
56. Assist for chest physiotherapy				
57. Perform active and passive exercises				
Orthopedic ward—1 week duration				
58. Assessment of orthopedic patients				
59. Assisting in the application of plaster cast				
60. Assisting in the removal of cast				
61. Assisting in applying skin traction				
62. Assisting in bucks extension traction				
63. Assisting in application of prosthesis				
64. Physiotherapy				
65. Crutch maneuvering technique				
66. Assisting for ambulation				
67. Care of amputated patient				
Communicable diseases ward/isolation ward—1 week duration				
68. Assessment of patient with communicable diseases				
69. Use of personal protective equipment (PPE) and barrier nursing techniques				

Procedure	*Date of demonstration*	*Teacher signature*	*Date of return demonstration*	*Supervisor signature*
70. Counseling of HIV/AIDS patient				
71. Counseling of patient and family members				
72. Health teaching on prevention of infectious diseases				
Emergency ward/casualty—1 week duration				
73. Practice triage				
74. Assist in emergency and disaster situations				
75. Provide first aid				
76. Perform ACLS/BLS				
77. Assist in legal documentation				
78. Assist in emergency procedures				
79. Counseling patient and family members in grief and bereavement				

Nursing Care Plan in Medical and Surgical Wards

Sl. No.	*Date*	*Details of care plan*	*Ward*	*Supervisor signature*
1.				
2.				
3.				
4.				

Case Study in Medical and Surgical Wards

Sl. No.	*Date*	*Details of case study*	*Ward*	*Supervisor signature*
1.				
2.				

Case Presentation in Medical and Surgical Wards

Sl. No.	*Date*	*Details of case presentation*	*Ward*	*Supervisor signature*
1.				
2.				

Drug Presentation in Medical and Surgical Wards

Sl. No.	*Date*	*Details of drugs*	*Ward*	*Supervisor signature*
1.				

Health Talks Performed in the Hospital

Sl. No.	*Date*	*Place*	*Topic*	*Group/individual*	*AV aids used*	*Supervisor signature*
1.						
2.						
3.						
4.						
5.						

Attendance in percentage (%):

Theory:

Practical:

Subject teachers **Class coordinator** **Principal**

1.
2.
3.
4.

MEDICAL SURGICAL NURSING PRACTICAL EXAMINATION

Signature of internal examiner **Signature of external examiner**

Date: **Date:**

Signature of internal examiner **Signature of external examiner**

Date: **Date:**

Signature of internal examiner **Signature of external examiner**

Date: **Date:**

MENTAL HEALTH NURSING

Placement: II Year—Clinical Hours: 320 (8 Weeks) and Internship: 96 hours (2 Weeks)

Procedure	*Date of demonstration*	*Teacher signature*	*Date of return demonstration*	*Supervisor signature*
Psychiatric OPD—1 week duration				
1. History taking				
2. Mental status examination—1				
3. Mental status examination—2				
4. Assist in psychometric assessment				
5. Counseling and educating patients and family members				
6. Observational report of OPD				
Child guidance clinic—1 week duration				
7. History taking				
8. Mental status examination				
9. Observe and assist for therapies				
10. Counsel family members and significant others				
11. Health education of family members and significant others				
12. Observational report of child guidance clinic				
Inpatient ward—6 weeks duration				
13. History taking				
14. Mental status examination—1				
15. Mental status examination—2				
16. Admission procedure				
17. Discharge procedure				
18. Process recording—1				
19. Process recording—2				
20. Case study				
21. Care plan				
22. Case presentation				
23. Assist and prepare for various therapies				
23.1. Electroconvulsive therapy				
23.2. Individual psychotherapy				
23.3. Behavior therapy				
23.4. Recreational therapy				
23.5. Occupational therapy				
24. Administration of psychotropic drugs				

Field Visits

Sl. No.	*Date*	*Visit*	*Institution address*	*Supervisor signature*
1.		Community mental health center		
2.		Half way home		
3.		Deaddiction center		
4.		Certified school		
5.		Old age home		

Observational Reports

Sl. No.	Details	Date of submission	Supervisor signature
1.	Observational report of psychiatric OPD		
2.	Observational report of child guidance clinic		
3.	Observational report of deaddiction center		
4.	Observational report of community mental health center		

Nursing Care Plan in Psychiatric Wards

Sl. No.	Date	Details of care plan/case study/case presentation	Ward	Supervisor signature
1.				
2.				
3.				

Drug Presentation in Psychiatric Wards

Sl. No.	Date	Details of drugs	Ward	Supervisor signature
1.				

Health Talks Performed in the Hospital

Sl. No.	Date	Place	Topic	Group/individual	AV aids used	Supervisor signature
1.						
2.						
3.						
4.						

Details of Psychiatric Nursing Clinical Postings

Name of the Mental Hospital/Nursing home:

Attendance in percentage (%):

Theory:

Practical:

Subject teachers **Class coordinator** **Principal**

1.
2.
3.

MENTAL HEALTH NURSING PRACTICAL EXAMINATION

Signature of internal examiner **Signature of external examiner**

Date: **Date:**

Signature of internal examiner **Signature of external examiner**

Date: **Date:**

Signature of internal examiner **Signature of external examiner**

Date: **Date:**

CHILD HEALTH NURSING

Placement: II Year—Clinical Hours: 320 (8 Weeks) and Internship: 96 Hours (2 Weeks)

Procedure	*Date of demonstration*	*Teacher signature*	*Date of return demonstration*	*Supervisor signature*
Pediatric medical ward—3 weeks duration				
1. **Assessment of sick child**				
1.1. Collect pediatric history				
1.2. Perform physical examination				
1.3. Growth and development assessment				
1.4. Nutritional assessment				
1.5. Anthropometric measurements				
1.6. Assessment of child				
2. **Administration of medications and injections**				
2.1. Oral				
2.2. Intramuscular				
2.3. Intravenous				
2.4. Subcutaneous				
2.5. Intradermal				
2.6. Topical				
2.7. Rectal				
3. **Calculation of fluid requirements**				
3.1. Preparing different strengths of IV fluids				
4. **Apply restraints**				
4.1. Mummy restraints				
4.2. Elbow restraints				
4.3. Crib with dome				
4.4. Jacket restraints				
4.5. Abdominal binder				
4.6. Mittens				
5. **Administer oxygen**				
6. **Feed children**				
6.1. Katori				
6.2. Spoon				
6.3. Palladi				
6.4. Nasogastric tube feeding				
6.5. Artificial feeding				
7. **Collect specimens for common investigations**				
7.1. Urine				
7.2. Blood				
7.3. Stool				
7.4. Sputum				
7.5. Throat swab				
8. Assist with common diagnostic procedures				

Procedure	*Date of demonstration*	*Teacher signature*	*Date of return demonstration*	*Supervisor signature*
9. Teach parents about balanced diet for children of different age groups: ➢ Newborn ➢ Infant ➢ Toddler ➢ Pre-schooler ➢ Schooler ➢ Adolescent				
10. **Newborn assessment**				
10.1. APGAR score assessment				
10.2. Gestational age assessment				
10.3. Assessment of reflexes				
10.4. Vital signs				
10.5. Weighing newborn				
10.6. Anthropometric measurements				
11. Nursing care of children with medical disorders				
12. Immediate newborn care				
13. Care of low birth weight baby				
14. Care of child in phototherapy				
15. Care of child in ICU				
16. Care of child on ventilator				
17. Oral rehydration therapy				
18. Feeding and weaning				
19. Play therapy				
20. **Check vital signs**				
20.1. Temperature				
20.2. Pulse				
20.3. Respiration				
20.4. Blood pressure				
21. Enema				
22. Insert suppositories				
Pediatric surgical ward—3 weeks duration				
23. **Care of child in surgical ward**				
23.1. Preoperative care				
23.2. Postoperative care				
24. Bowel wash				
25. **Care of ostomies**				
25.1. Colostomy				
25.2. Ureterostomy				
25.3. Gastrostomy				
25.4. Enterostomy				
25.5. Irrigations				
26. Urinary catheterization				
27. Maintaining urinary drainage				
28. **Feeding**				
28.1. Nasogastric				

Procedure	Date of demonstration	Teacher signature	Date of return demonstration	Supervisor signature
28.2. Gastrostomy				
28.3. Jejunostomy				
29. Care of surgical wound				
29.1. Dressing				
29.2. Suture removal				
Pediatric OPD/immunization/well baby clinic/adolescent clinic—2 weeks duration				
30. Assessment of children				
30.1. Health assessment				
30.2. Developmental assessment				
30.3. Anthropometric assessment				
31. Administering immunization				
32. Health/nutritional education				

Observational Reports

Sl. No.	Report	Date of submission	Signature supervisor
1.	Observational report of newborn		
2.	Observational report of newborn		

Nursing Care Plan/Case Study/Case Presentation in Pediatric Wards

Sl. No.	Date	Details of care plan/case study/case presentation	Ward	Supervisor signature
1.				
2.				
3.				
4.				

Drug Presentation in Pediatric Wards

Sl. No.	Date	Details of drugs	Ward	Supervisor signature
1.				

Health Talks Performed in the Pediatric Wards/OPD

Sl. No.	Date	Place	Topic	Group/individual	AV aids used	Supervisor signature
1.						
2.						

Attendance in percentage (%):

Theory:

Practical:

Subject teachers **Class coordinator** **Principal**

1.
2.
3.
4.

CHILD HEALTH NURSING PRACTICAL EXAMINATION

Signature of internal examiner **Signature of external examiner**

Date: **Date:**

Signature of internal examiner **Signature of external examiner**

Date: **Date:**

Signature of internal examiner **Signature of external examiner**

Date: **Date:**

SECOND YEAR EXAMINATION RESULTS

Name of the student: Month and year of passing:

Register No:

Hall ticket No:

Subject	*Type of assessment*	*Max. Marks*	*Marks obtained in first attempt*	*Marks obtained in second attempt*	*Marks obtained in third attempt*
PAPER – I Medical surgical nursing – I	Internal	25			
	Board/Council	75			
	Total	**100**			
PAPER – II Medical surgical nursing – II	Internal	25			
	Board/Council	75			
	Total	**100**			
PAPER – III Mental health nursing	Internal	25			
	Board/Council	75			
	Total	**100**			
PAPER – IV Child health nursing	Internal	25			
	Board/Council	75			
	Total	**100**			
PRACTICAL – I Medical surgical nursing	Internal	50			
	Board/Council	50			
	Total	**100**			
PRACTICAL – II Child health nursing	Internal	50			
	Board/Council	50			
	Total	**100**			
PRACTICAL – III Mental health nursing	Internal	50			
	Board/Council	50			
	Total	**100**			

Note: Minimum pass percentage—50% in each subject

THIRD YEAR

DETAILS OF COURSE INSTRUCTION (THEORY AND PRACTICAL)

Sl. No.	*Subjects*	*Hours prescribed by INC*	*Completed hours*	*Name of the teacher*	*Teacher signature*
		THEORY–PART I			
1.	Midwifery and gynecological nursing	140			
2.	Community health nursing – II	90			
3.	Co-curricular activities	10			
	Total	**240**			
		THEORY–PART II: Integrated Supervised Internship			
4.	Nursing education	20			
5.	Introduction to research and statistics	30			
6.	Professional trends and adjustments	30			
7.	Nursing administration and ward management	40			
	Total	**120**			
		PRACTICAL			
1.	Midwifery and gynecological nursing	560 (14 weeks)			
2.	Community health nursing – II	160 (4 weeks)			
	Total Hours (weeks)	**720 (18 weeks)**			

LIST OF THIRD YEAR ASSIGNMENTS

Maternity and gynaecological ward	*Community health nursing*
• Nursing care plan—3 • Case study—2 • Case presentation—2 • Drug study—2	• Daily diary—urban and rural • Health talk—2 each in urban and rural • Family health nursing care plan—2 each in urban and rural • Group project—1 each in urban and rural

In addition to above, each student shall maintain a procedure book and midwifery case book signed by the supervisor and principal to be submitted to the examiner.

MIDWIFERY AND GYNECOLOGICAL NURSING

Placement: III Year—Clinical Hours: 560 (14 Weeks) and Internship Hours: 384 (15 Weeks)

Procedure	*Date of demonstration*	*Teacher signature*	*Date of return demonstration*	*Supervisor signature*
Antenatal clinic/ward—2 weeks duration				
1. Diagnose pregnancy using pregnancy kit (preg-card)				
2. Antenatal history taking				
3. Physical examination				
4. **Antenatal abdominal examination**				
4.1. Inspection				
4.2. Palpation				
4.3. Auscultation				
5. Breast examination				
6. Recording weight				
7. Recording blood pressure				
8. Hemoglobin estimation				
9. Urine test for sugar				
10. Urine test for albumin				
11. Immunization				
12. Assessment of risk status				
13. Care of antenatal mother with high risk pregnancy				
14. Antenatal counseling on diet and exercises				
15. Maintenance of antenatal records				
16. Skilled birth attendant (SBA) module				
Labor room—4 weeks duration				
17. Assessment of women in labor				
18. Vaginal examination and its interpretation				
19. Monitor women in labor using partograph				
20. Administration of uterotonic drugs—oxytocin, misoprostol				
21. Administration of magnesium sulfate				
22. Care for women in labor				
23. Setting up labor unit including newborn corner				
24. Conducting normal delivery including active management of third stage of labor (AMTSL)				
25. **Immediate newborn assessment**				
25.1. APGAR score assessment				
25.2. Gestational age assessment				
25.3. Assessment of reflexes				
25.4. Vital signs				
25.5. Weighing newborn				
25.6. Anthropometric measurements				
25.7. Examination for birth defects				

Procedure	*Date of demonstration*	*Teacher signature*	*Date of return demonstration*	*Supervisor signature*
26. **Provide essential newborn care**				
26.1. Mummification				
26.2. Bonding and rooming in				
26.3. Initiating breastfeeding				
Operation theater—1 week duration				
27. Preparation for cesarean section and other surgical procedures				
28. Assisting in cesarean section				
29. Preparation and assisting in Medical Termination of Pregnancy (MTP) procedure				
30. Preparation and assisting for tubectomy				
Postnatal ward—3 weeks duration				
31. Examination and assessment of mother and the baby				
32. Identification of deviations				
33. Care of postnatal mother and baby				
34. Perineal care				
35. Breast care				
36. Lactation management				
37. Breastfeeding				
38. Kangaroo mother care (KMC)				
39. Immunization				
40. Teach postnatal mother on mother craft				
41. Teach postnatal mother on postnatal care and exercises				
42. Teach postnatal mother on immunization				
43. Assessment of episiotomy by REEDA scale				
44. Care of high risk postnatal mother				
Newborn intensive care unit (NICU)—2 weeks duration				
45. Newborn assessment				
46. Admission of neonates				
47. **Feeding high risk newborn**				
47.1. Katori				
47.2. Spoon				
47.3. Paladai				
47.4. Tube feeding				
47.5, Total parental nutrition				
48. **Thermal management of newborns**				
48.1. Kangaroo mother care				
48.2. Care of baby in radiant warmer				
48.3. Care of baby in incubator				
49. Monitor and care of neonates				
50. Administration of medications				
51. Intravenous therapy				
52. Assist in diagnostic procedures				
53. Assist in exchange transfusion				
54. Care of baby on ventilator				

Procedure	Date of demonstration	Teacher signature	Date of return demonstration	Supervisor signature
55. Care of baby in phototherapy				
56. Implement infection control protocols				
57. Health education and counseling of parents				
58. Maintenance of records and reports				
Family welfare clinic—1 week duration				
59. Family planning counseling techniques				
60. Insertion of intrauterine contraceptive device (IUCD)				
61. Teaching on use of different family planning methods				
62. Arrange and assist with family planning operations				
62.1. Tubectomy				
62.2. Vasectomy				
63. Maintenance of records and reports				
Gynecology ward—1 week duration				
64. Assisting with gynecological examination				
65. Assisting and performing diagnostic and therapeutic procedures				
66. Teaching women on breast self-examination (BSE)				
67. Health education on perineal hygiene and prevention of sexually transmitted infections				
68. Pre and postoperative care of women undergoing gynecological surgeries				
69. Menopause counseling				

Essential Requirements

Sl. No.	Assignment	Number of requirements	Teacher signature
1.	Conduct antenatal examinations	10	
2.	Perform per vaginal examinations	05	
3.	Conduct normal deliveries	20	
4.	Perform and suture episiotomy	05	
5.	Resuscitate newborn	05	
6.	Witness abnormal deliveries	05	
7.	Assist with cesarean section	02	
8.	Provide postnatal care to mothers and babies	20	
9.	IUCD insertion	05	
10.	Family planning counseling	02	
11.	Menopause counseling	01	

Observational Reports

Sl. No.	Details	Date of submission	Supervisor signature
1.			
2.			

Nursing Care Plans in Maternity and Gynecological Ward

Sl. No.	Date	Details of care plan	Ward	Supervisor signature
1.				
2.				
3.				

Case Studies in Maternity and Gynecological Ward

Sl. No.	Date	Details of case study	Ward	Supervisor signature
1.				
2.				

Case Presentation in Maternity and Gynecological Ward

Sl. No.	Date	Details of case presentation	Ward	Supervisor signature
1.				
2.				

Drug Study in Maternity and Gynecological Wards

Sl. No.	Date	Details of drugs	Ward	Supervisor signature
1.				
2.				

Health Talks Performed in Maternity and Gynecological Wards

Sl. No.	Date	Place	Topic	Group/individual	AV aids used	Supervisor signature
1.						
2.						
3.						

Attendance in percentage (%):

Theory:

Practical:

Subject teachers	**Class coordinator**	**Principal**
1.		
2.		
3.		
4.		

MIDWIFERY AND GYNECOLOGICAL NURSING PRACTICAL EXAMINATION

Signature of internal examiner	**Signature of external examiner**
Date:	**Date:**
Signature of internal examiner	**Signature of external examiner**
Date:	**Date:**
Signature of internal examiner	**Signature of external examiner**
Date:	**Date:**

COMMUNITY HEALTH NURSING – II

Placement: III Year—Practical Hours: 160 (4 Weeks) and Internship Hours: 288 (6 Weeks)

Procedure	*Date of demonstration*	*Teacher signature*	*Date of return demonstration*	*Supervisor signature*
Urban /rural posting—4 weeks duration				
1. **Mapping the field area**				
1.1. Rural				
1.2. Urban				
2. **Assisting in survey activities**				
2.1. Community health survey in rural area				
2.2. Community health survey in urban area				
2.3. Identification of community needs				
3. **Organization and conduct of home visits**				
3.1. Build up and maintain rapport with family				
3.2. Demonstrate bag technique				
3.3. Assessment of family environment				
3.4. Housing/sanitary condition				
3.5. Health assessment of family				
3.6. Nutritional assessment of individuals				
4. **Identification and listing of health needs**				
4.1. Antenatal mother				
4.2. Postnatal mother				
4.3. Infant				
4.4. Toddler				
4.5. Pre-schooler				
4.6. School age child				
4.7. Adolescent				
4.8. Adult				
4.9. Old age person				
4.10. Sick person if any				
4.11. Listing the health needs of the family				
5. **Providing nursing care at home as per standing orders**				
5.1. Antenatal mother				
5.2. Postnatal mother				
5.3. Patient with tuberculosis				
5.4. Patient with leprosy				
5.5. Patient with STD/AIDS/HIV positive				
5.6. Planning and carrying out treatment for minor ailments				
6. **Providing prescribed treatment at home setting**				
6.1. Oral medication				
6.2. Intramuscular injection				
6.3. Subcutaneous injection				
6.4. Intravenous Infusion				
6.5. Instillation of eye drops				
6.6. Instillation of ear drops				

Procedure	*Date of demonstration*	*Teacher signature*	*Date of return demonstration*	*Supervisor signature*
6.7. Instillation of nose drops				
6.8. Identifying the need for referral and make referrals				
6.9. Planning and conducting individual health education on identified needs				
6.10. Planning and conducting group health education				
6.11. Maintaining family folders				
7. Assisting for set up of clinics in the community				
7.1. Antenatal				
7.2. Postnatal				
7.3. Under five				
7.4. Sneha				
7.5. Non-communicable disease				
7.6. Geriatric				
7.7. Immunization				
7.8. Family planning				
7.9. School health				
8. Assisting in health center activities—Subcenter, Primary Health Center (PHC), Community Health Center (CHC)				
8.1. Health assessment at OPD				
8.2. Assisting in immunization activities				
8.3. Administration of medications				
8.4. Wound care/dressing				
8.5. Antenatal care				
8.6. Conducting normal deliveries				
8.7. Newborn care				
8.8. Postnatal care				
8.9. Collection and record of vital health statistics				
8.10. Assisting in activities related to National Health Program				
9. Assisting in family planning/welfare activities				
9.1. Oral pills				
9.2. Insertion of copper T				
9.3. Medical termination of pregnancy				
9.4. Tubectomy				
9.5. Vasectomy				
9.6. Educating on family welfare activities				
10. Maintenance of records and reports				
10.1. Birth register				
10.2. Death register				
10.3. Immunization register				
10.4. Antenatal register				
10.5. Postnatal register				
10.6. Family planning register				
10.7. Stock register				

Procedure	Date of demonstration	Teacher signature	Date of return demonstration	Supervisor signature
10.8. Morbidity register				
11. Conducting health education				
11.1. Conducting need based individual health education				
11.2. Group health education				
11.3. Mass health education				
12. School health program				
12.1. Health assessment of school children				
12.2. Treatment for minor ailments				
12.3. Health education				
12.4. Referral services				

Observational Visits

Sl. No.	Date	Visit	Supervisor signature
1.		Municipal corporation	
2.		Panchayat office	
3.		Health block office/District health office	
4.		Homes for differently abled children	
5.		Old age home	
6.		Community health center	
7.		Family planning association	
8.		Voluntary health agencies	
9.		Community rehabilitation center	
10.		Industry	

Assignments Performed in the Community

Sl. No.	Assignment	Date	Area/House address	Supervisor signature
1.	Family care plan (name of the family) 1. 2. 3. 4.			
2.	Daily diary	Submission date:		

Group Project Work in Community

Sl. No.	Topic	No. of group members	Date of submission	Supervisor signature
1.				

School Health Program

Sl. No.	Name of the school	No. of children	Date	Supervisor signature
1.				

Health Talks Performed in Rural and Urban Community

Sl. No.	*Date*	*Place*	*Topic*	*Group/individual*	*AV aids used*	*Supervisor signature*
1.						
2.						
3.						
4.						

Attendance in percentage (%):

Theory:

Practical:

Subject teachers **Class coordinator** **Principal**

1.
2.
3.
4.

COMMUNITY HEALTH NURSING – II PRACTICAL EXAMINATION

Signature of internal examiner **Signature of external examiner**

Date: **Date:**

Signature of internal examiner **Signature of external examiner**

Date: **Date:**

Signature of internal examiner **Signature of external examiner**

Date: **Date:**

INTERNSHIP PERIOD

NURSING EDUCATION

Placement: III Year (Part II)—20 Hours

Procedure	*Date of demonstration*	*Teacher signature*	*Date of return demonstration*	*Supervisor signature*
1. **Methods of classroom teaching**				
1.1. Lecture				
1.2. Group discussion				
1.3. Symposium				
1.4. Seminar				
1.5. Demonstration				
2. **Methods of teaching in clinical area**				
2.1. Bedside teaching				
2.2. Case discussion				
2.3. Nursing rounds				
2.4. Nursing conference				
2.5. Process recording				
3. **Preparation of plans**				
3.1. Course plan				
3.2. Unit plan				
3.3. Lesson plan				
4. **Preparation of audio-visual aids**				
4.1. Charts				
4.2. Flash cards				
4.3. Transparencies				
4.4. Models				
4.5. Posters				
4.6. PowerPoint				

Observational Reports

Sl. No.	*Details*	*Date of submission*	*Supervisor signature*
1.	State Nursing Council		
2.	Local TNAI office		

Attendance in percentage (%):

Theory:

Practical:

Subject teachers **Class coordinator** **Principal**

1.

2.

NURSING ADMINISTRATION AND WARD MANAGEMENT

Placement: III Year (Part II)—40 Hours

Procedure	*Date of demonstration*	*Teacher signature*	*Date of return demonstration*	*Supervisor signature*
1. **Preparation of organizational chart**				
1.1. Nursing service department				
1.2. Nursing school				
2. **Preparation of duty rosters**				
2.1. Nursing officers				
2.2. Nursing supervisors				
2.3. Students				
2.4. Class D staff				
3. **Indenting process**				
3.1. Drugs				
3.2. Supplies				
3.3. Equipment				
3.4. Maintaining drug inventory				
3.5. Preparation of requisition letters for repair and replacements				
4. **Maintaining records**				
4.1. Admission register				
4.2. Discharge register				
4.3. Drug register				
4.4. Census record				
4.5. Day report				
4.6. Night report				
4.7. Rounds register				
4.8. Staff attendance register				
4.9. Leave register				
4.10. Biomedical waste management register				
4.11. Incident report register				
4.12. Medicolegal register				
4.13. Service register				
4.14. Death register				
4.15. Birth register				
4.16. Drug indent register				
4.17. CSSD register				
4.18. Inventory register				
4.19. Lenin register				
5. **Preparation of job descriptions**				
5.1. Nursing superintendent				
5.2. Nursing supervisor				
5.3. Nursing officer				
5.4. Principal				
5.5. Vice-principal				
5.6. Senior nursing tutor				

Procedure	*Date of demonstration*	*Teacher signature*	*Date of return demonstration*	*Supervisor signature*
5.7. Junior nursing tutor				
5.8. Clinical instructor				
6. Organization/assisting in organization of				
6.1. Orientation program to new staff				
6.2. Staff developmental programs				
6.3. Staff welfare programs				
6.4. Clinical presentations				
7. Preparation of tools				
7.1. Performance appraisal for staff				
7.2. Evaluation tool for students				
7.3. Evaluation tool for patient care				
7.4. Patient care protocols				

Attendance in percentage (%):

Theory:

Practical:

Subject teachers **Class coordinator** **Principal**

1.
2.
3.
4.

THIRD YEAR EXAMINATION RESULTS

Name of the student: Month and year of passing:

Register No:

Hall ticket No:

Subject	*Type of assessment*	*Max. Marks*	*Marks obtained in first attempt*	*Marks obtained in second attempt*	*Marks obtained in third attempt*
PAPER – I Midwifery and gynecological nursing	Internal	25			
	Board/Council	75			
	Total	**100**			
PAPER – II Community health nursing – II	Internal	25			
	Board/Council	75			
	Total	**100**			
PRACTICAL – I Midwifery	Internal	50			
	Board/Council	50			
	Total	**100**			
PRACTICAL – II Community health nursing	Internal	50			
	Board/Council	50			
	Total	**100**			

Note: Minimum pass percentage—50% in each subject